The Truth about Sugar Detox

Why a Sugar Detox Works

By: Amy Zulpa

TABLE OF CONTENTS

PUBLISHERS NOTES

Disclaimer

This publication is intended to provide helpful and informative material. It is not intended to diagnose, treat, cure, or prevent any health problem or condition, nor is intended to replace the advice of a physician. No action should be taken solely on the contents of this book. Always consult your physician or qualified health-care professional on any matters regarding your health and before adopting any suggestions in this book or drawing inferences from it.

The author and publisher specifically disclaim all responsibility for any liability, loss or risk, personal or otherwise, which is incurred as a consequence, directly or indirectly, from the use or application of any contents of this book.

Any and all product names referenced within this book are the trademarks of their respective owners. None of these owners have sponsored, authorized, endorsed, or approved this book.

Always read all information provided by the manufacturers' product labels before using their products. The author and publisher are not responsible for claims made by manufacturers.

© 2014

Manufactured in the United States of America

DEDICATION

This book is dedicated to my parents.

CHAPTER 1- WHAT IS THE SUGAR DETOX ALL ABOUT?

Sugar, how sweet it is and dangerous to your health. Sixty nine percent of Americans are overweight. We can trace this problem to our craving for sugar. We eat an average of 19 teaspoons of sugar a day. The recommended amount is only six teaspoons per day. In one year we consume 70 pounds of sugar. The excess consumption is so large that some are calling for sugar to be labeled a "controlled" substance, limiting intake to 31 pounds per year. There is a link between sugar intake and diabetes. Officials estimate that one in three persons will have diabetes by the year 2050.

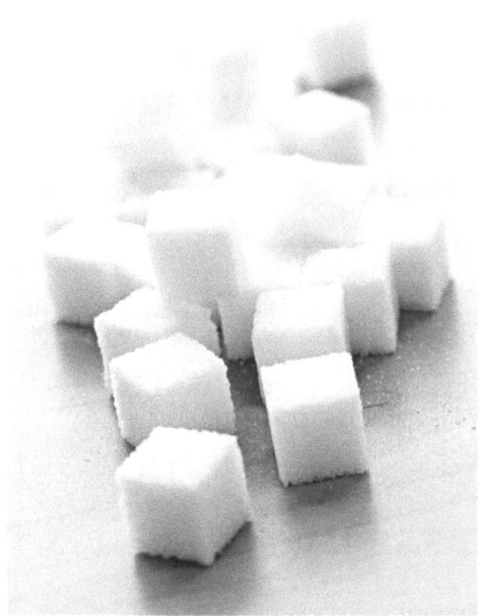

Most Americans have programmed their taste buds to crave sugar from their first bottle of milk. Milk contains lactose that is sugar. So we can see how easy it is to develop a sugar addiction. Add to this our change in lifestyle over the past two decades. We eat our more often. Most restaurants serve up oversize portions with usually potatoes or fries. Then we top off these "wonderful" meals with the most delicious desserts on earth, all loaded with sugar. With two workers per household in many families, take-out has become a dinner staple. Pizza is a favorite. If it's not take-out, we often see the family eating at a fast food restaurant; and the soda, forget about it. We not only have a normal size cup but now the norm is a gigantic cup, loaded to the max with sugar. So if it's not the food it's the drink that is putting us on the fast track to sugar addiction.

Sugar fuels every cell in the brain. It creates a quick high by drawing Insulin from the pancreas. The insulin processes the sugar quickly. When the high disappears our blood sugar gets low again, setting a new craving in motion. This reinforces the craving and a sugar addiction is now growing stronger. Some researchers compare sugar addiction to cocaine addiction.

Meanwhile a group of scientific studies have identified the links between sugar and several diseases including diabetes, heart disease, obesity, high blood pressure, high cholesterol, Alzheimer's and cataracts. These studies have led us to develop ways of reducing sugar consumption. One method is to "detox" or rid the body of sugar completely. Some advocates recommend a slow approach by eliminating sugar intake over several weeks by gradually dropping sugary foods from our diet.

Others advocate a "cold turkey" approach of cutting out all sugars from the start. There are several sugar detox programs. These are not diets. They differ in that they have a single goal and that is to eliminate sugar completely and permanently from our diet. However they do end up eliminating virtually all sugars and carbohydrates, replacing them with protein and some sugars from fruits. Nuts, lean chicken, salads and fish are recommended.

These detox programs vary in length from a three day detox to longer 21 days to 30 days. They also vary in the exact foods you can eat. For example, one three day detox is the most radical with no dairy, no fruit except lemon and lime, no wheat and starches and no added sugars. The 21 day detox is the most flexible. Both Facebook and Pinterest have descriptions, recipes, and feedback from other viewers.

The 21 day program involves removing all sugar and simple carbohydrates from your diet and removing all foods on the "avoid" list. If you fail this detox for just one day you must start over at day one. So, if you mess up on day 19, you must start over again. Some of the comments on Facebook are quite interesting. One woman said that she treats sugar detox just like she did her alcohol addition, one day at a time. She says that she stopped "cold turkey" and now has virtually no craving for sugar. The 30 day program is similar, just spread out over a longer period.

Your food shopping becomes more challenging. You must read the labels carefully, especially for any packaged foods. They almost always contain sugar. Cereals, cookies, pastries, breads, fruit juices and the most dangerous of all, "soda," just to name a few, all contain sugar. Then you must be on the lookout for "hidden" or sleeper sugars, sugars that are disguised under other names. These include agave nectar, brown rice syrup, glucose, molasses, lactose, evaporated sugar cane, ketchup, high fructose corn syrup, dextrose, sucrose, BBQ sauces, bread, salad dressings, pasta sauce and flavored coffees. You also have the whole group of artificial sugar sweeteners. Splenda is from a plant grown in Paraguay or Brazil. It is 500 times sweeter than sugar. Agave is another natural sweetener that comes from the blue agave cactus.

Persons that have gone through a sugar detox have stated that they experience fat loss, less bloating, clearer skin, increase in taste for healthier foods, regular bowel movements increased energy, sense of well being, elevated mood, lower cholesterol and better sleep.

Whether or not we choose a sugar detox, the path is clear. We must consciously decide to cut our sugar intake. Not doing so will put our overall health at risk.

CHAPTER 2- WHAT ARE THE ADVANTAGES OF A SUGAR DETOX?

Many people nowadays are starting to care more and more about their health. They realize that the things that they eat have a huge impact on how they feel. More and more people are making the decision to cut out foods that can harm the body, and to only put things in their bodies that are going to be beneficial. Sugar is one of those things that people love, but sugar, in the end, is just empty calories.

Many studies have proven that sugar actually has an addictive component that makes people want to keep eating it once they start. Many people do not realize that sugar has this addictive power, and because of that, they fall victim to its snare. There have been a great number of people that have decided to do a sugar detox. It may sound weird that people want to have a detox of sugar, but in reality a lot of sugar in a person's body can do a lot more damage than many people would imagine.

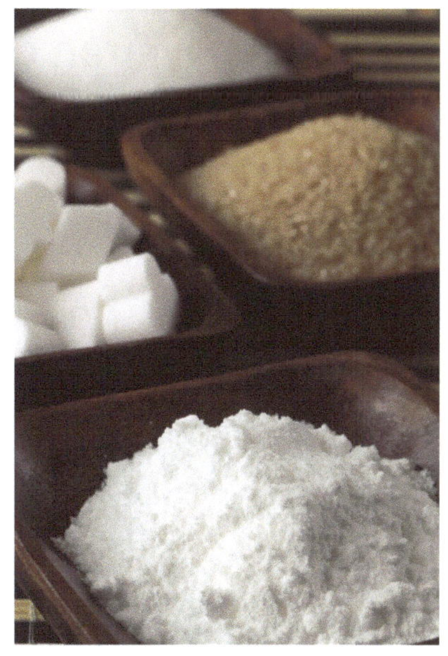

Why Detox?

The average American eats about 150 pounds of sugar a year. That is an astonishing figure when a person takes their own weight into account. For an average woman that would mean that she eats more sugar in a year than she weighs. One of the many bad things about sugar is that it is just empty calories. If a person eats fruits, vegetables, meats and cheeses, they are eating things that give them calories, but at the same time, they are eating things that give them nutrition as well. When it comes to sugar, a person does not receive any nutrition or anything positive at all, all they get is calories in their bodies, with no benefit.

More than ever, people that eat the North and South American diet are getting diagnosed with diabetes. There are two types of diabetes. One is completely hereditary and the other is based on diet and sugar. When a person eats too much sugar they could trigger a release of the hormone insulin. A person's insulin can go up very high, and if that happens over an extended period of time a person could get diabetes.

Diabetes is a very serious disease and if it is not taken care of it can cause blindness, loss of limbs, heart attacks, strokes, and death. Too much sugar can make a person feel happy and high at first, but after a while a high sugar diet can cause a person to crash and to feel like their bodies are sluggish. It has also been proven that a diet that is high in sugar can cause a person to have high cholesterol and high blood pressure.

How to Do a Sugar Cleanse

First, it is important to determine the amount of time that you want to spend doing a sugar detox. Many people decide to just do the cleanse for a week or so, but the best type of sugar cleanse usually will last for at least 21 days. The first thing that needs to be eliminated is sodas, and any other fruit drink that is not 100 percent juice. Other things like processed foods, candy and any other type of food that contain sugar need to be eliminated from the diet. That even includes condiments. It is important to check labels of the foods that are eaten. If the food contains fructose, sorbitol, cane juice or maltose, it should be avoided. Of course if any type of sugar is in on the label it should not be consumed.

How To Eat On the Sugar Cleanse

Eating food on the sugar cleanse is not as hard as some people think. There are great websites that give ideas of meals and snack plans that a person can eat in order to avoid eating sugar. The first important thing to eat is protein. Protein packs a punch to blood sugar, it helps blood sugar to be stable and also it can prevent a person from having strong sugar cravings.

There are great things to snack on that are found in nature and that do not have any sugar. Fresh vegetables and fruits are great for the body, and they are perfectly fine to eat on the sugar detox. Whole grains and legumes are also good to eat on this meal plan. Salads are great to eat on the sugar detox. There are literally thousands of different ways that a person can make a salad. There is not even really a need to eat sweetened salad dressing, because it is easy to make a great dressing with just vinegar and olive oil.

Why So Beneficial

The benefits of the sugar cleanse are many and abounding. First a person's blood sugar, and cholesterol will go down greatly. A person will feel more refreshed and alert during the day. They will have more focus and they will feel like they have a lot more energy. Going off of sugar can help in many other ways as well. It can help a person to get a good night's sleep, and if a person is suffering from any kind of body or skin inflammation or irritation, they will soon see that their skin problem will disappear completely, or get a lot better. A person will also see that their skin is glowing more and that their eyes will look a lot less puffy. Perhaps the best thing out of all of the rest is that a person will lose weight on this cleanse.

There are so many benefits to doing a sugar cleanse. It is actually one of the most simple cleanses to do, but the benefits are enormous. Once a person does the sugar cleanse, they may also begin to notice that they no longer need that much sugar in their daily diets anymore.

CHAPTER 3- STARTING A SUGAR DETOX-THE MAIN STEPS

If you've made the decision to reduce the amount of sugar in your diet, chances are your detox will result in you having more energy and mental clarity. Excess sugar has the ability to make you sluggish and decrease concentration. When you don't have enough fiber in your diet, the body will also turn most of the sugar you eat into fat, which leads to unwanted weight gain. Once you're ready to start your sugar detox, here are the important steps to follow.

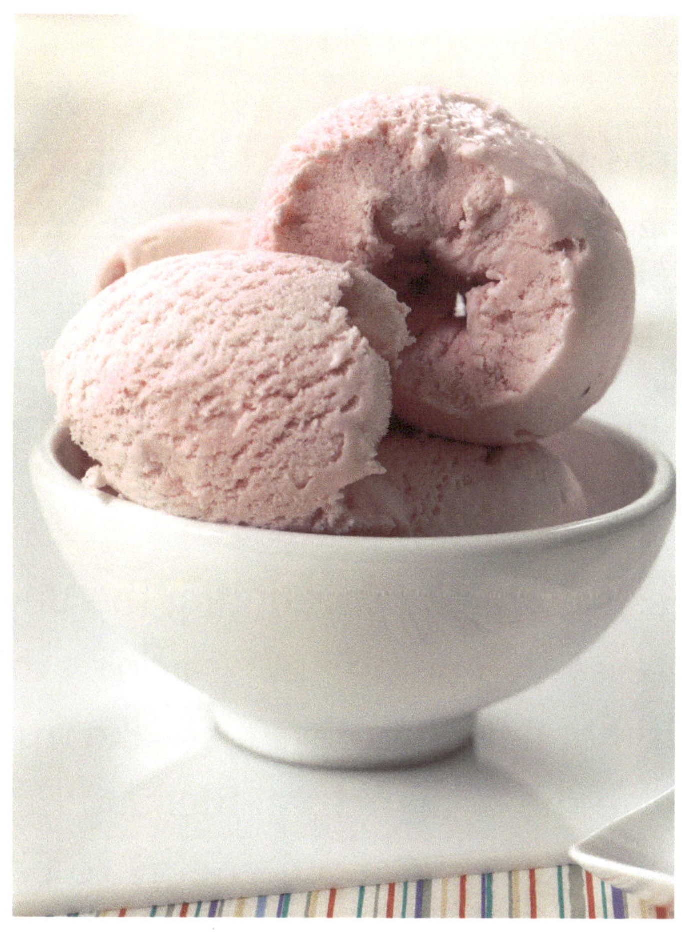

Pinpoint Your Cravings

It's important to know exactly which sugary foods are a temptation for you in order to make your sugar detox successful. When you make the conscious decision to give up processed sugar, your cravings for the foods your body is used to eating will likely get much stronger. If donuts are your favorite breakfast food, replace them with whole grain muffins sweetened with fruit juice. If you love having a piece of cake or pie after dinner, try eating your favorite piece of fruit for dessert instead. This way, you're still getting sugar, but in a much healthier form, and you'll be satisfying your hunger.

Eat More Often

One of the reasons your body may crave sugar often is because you're not eating enough. The body needs energy to function, and uses sugar to create glycogen and glucose, which is why you feel especially hyper or energetic after eating sugar. However, you'll likely experience a crash in your energy after an hour or two if you're eating processed sugar.

Eating several healthy small meals during the day will supply the body with necessary energy by raising the metabolism. Consuming foods that have natural sugars like fruits, whole grains and vegetables give the body natural fuel and help to burn fat at a faster rate. You'll also have more energy to complete tasks at work or maintain a rigorous exercise workout program.

Snacks on Fruits and Nuts

Snacks like nuts and fruits will help to decrease your desire to eat unhealthy sugary foods. Fruits won't raise your blood sugar level too high, and the natural sugar or fructose in fruit can satisfy your sweet tooth while helping you avoid an energy crash. Nuts are also a low-glycemic food that will supply the body with protein, which helps you maintain mental focus throughout the day and stick to your weight loss goals.

Cut Out Soft Drinks

Sodas are a major source of sugar, and soft drinks that contain both caffeine and high amounts of sugar are likely to make you more alert for a short period of time before making you feel exhausted. When you're detoxing your body from sugar, it's important to stay away from sodas, even the diet varieties, to sustain increased energy levels throughout the day. There are also hidden dangers in sugar free sodas; in fact, a study at Harvard Medical School reports that women who drink two or more diet colas daily are 30% more likely to have kidney problems.

If you consume sodas as a way to get a pick-me-up throughout the day, try alternatives like chicory coffee or green tea sweetened a healthy type of sugar like Stevia leaf or organic honey. These beverages are also ideal to consume in the mornings instead of prepared coffee drinks that are often laden with lots of sugar in the form of actual sugar, milk or flavored syrups.

Eliminate Simple Carbohydrates

Remember, sugars are also in foods that don't taste sweet. Simple carbohydrates like white bread and rice, as well as processed pasts are also forms of sugar that can cause the same effects in the body as cookies and pastries. Choose carbohydrates that are low on the glycemic index for your sugar detox, such as brown rice, whole grain bread (which is not the same as multi-grain bread), and whole grain pasta. These foods will keep you full for a longer period of time. The fiber in these complex carbohydrates will also keep the body from turning the natural sugar in the food into fat.

Determine the Reason for Your Cravings

Finally, figure out the real reason why your body is excessively craving sugar. Even though you've determine which foods you're drawn to, you may not entire understand why you love to eat them so much.

If your adrenal glands are overworking themselves, you're naturally going to crave sugar to try to restore the energy levels in your body. If you've been under a lot of stress lately, your body is producing more cortisol, or 'stress hormone,' which directly contributes to sugar cravings. Desiring sugar throughout the day can also be the result of Candida overgrowth in the body. Excessive Candida can also be characterized by symptoms like excessive eating, chronic fatigue, hormonal imbalance and mental fogginess.

To truly detox from sugar and prevent filling your body from sugary substances again after your cleanse, treat the underlying cause of your cravings while eliminating sugar from your diet. Take probiotics to balance the Candida in your body or take herbs like alfalfa to boost the health of your adrenal glands.

To reduce stress, stick to a regular exercise program to increase your endorphins. Your workout plan can be as simple as walking a mile or two in the evenings after dinner or participating in a yoga class to help clear your mind of negative thoughts while reducing body fat.

CHAPTER 4- HOW THE BODY HANDLES A SUGAR DETOX

It may not be something that you want to hear, but often times the things that our body enjoys the most are the things that are the worst for us. A perfect example of this is with sugar. Whether you are someone who enjoys drinking sugary soda, eating candy bars, or simply overloading everything you eat with sweet ingredients, the sugar in your life can have hazardous effects.

However, one way to get rid of this is with a sugar detox and while a sugar detox may be a bit extreme for some, it is a great option for those looking to clean up their body. Here is a look at how you handle a sugar detox and what to expect.

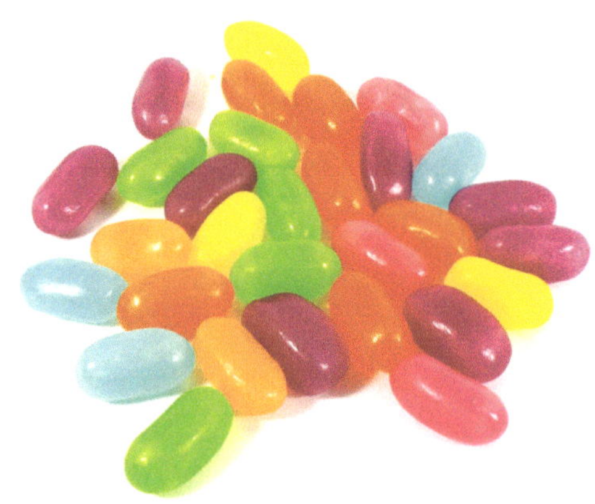

At First

When you first decide to stop making sugar part of your daily routine, you may not even notice at first. Most likely, your body will still have plenty of sugar and it will use those remaining deposits as much as possible because it isn't getting refills of new amounts of sugar. However, you may also notice that your body begins to feel a bit sluggish and that you have less energy. This is typically because sugar gives you unhealthy and unnatural spikes of energy. When you continually supplement your body with this, you are simply giving energy boosts that immediately come crashing down. When going through a sugar detox, you won't have as elevated of highs in terms of energy, and therefore you'll notice drastic amounts of lost energy. But don't worry, it's only temporary and it'll start to work itself out.

And Then

They say that things have to get worse, before they start getting better. Well, this is typically the case with the sugar detox. You'll likely notice that the energy you have decreases even more. Those sugar deposits that your body was feeding off of in the last section have likely all begun to deplete and your body is confused where all of the sugar has gone. While the body continues to search for sugar, it will burn energy in other ways, which is going to be the reason that you feel so sluggish and down.

Not only will your body desire sugar, but your brain will also begin to wonder where it has all gone. Your brain works very differently when it has sugar in the mix. But when it doesn't, it can have a hard time trying to refocus things in a way that is natural. With the combination of desire from your body and brain, it's very likely that this is when the sugar cravings will kick in.

Your mouth will water over the idea of a soda or a piece of chocolate. You may even think that just a bit of sugar is a fine way of getting past it. However, you have already broken past the hardest part and now is the time to stay strong. By not putting sugar back into your body, you will continue riding the wave of momentum that you have for during your sugar detox.

In order to combat the sugar cravings that you have, figure out ways to help motivate you even further. You can rely on a support system that consists of family or friends, or you can find a new hobby like going to the gym or picking up a musical instrument. The more that you can you're your mind off of sugar, the better you'll be at avoiding those cravings.

Until

Then, one day you'll wake up and feel different. You won't feel sluggish or drained, but rather energetic and reinvigorated. It's likely that you'll feel clear minded and have a refreshing feeling of your surroundings. This is when you have broken through and your body is adjusting to not depending on sugar. Not only has all of the sugar gone through your body, but your brain is also becoming more adjusted to the sugar-less desires. Overall, your system starts working better and you start feeling more healthy.

Better yet, you might also notice that when you hope on the scale that you are weighing less. It's quite possible that you may even look in the mirror and notice less love-handles and more definition. Once the sugar is gone, your body begins burning fat, rather than the sugar itself. This will result in you losing weight and looking and feeling a lot better. And if you adhered to the advice above by picking up a gym membership to keep your mind off sugar, you can bet that your results will be even better. The more that you do to benefit your body, the better you will feel once you break through the sugar detox barrier.

Keep Going

Going through a sugar detox deserves a big pat on the back. However, not falling back into the same traps and lifestyle choices is what you will find to be the real challenge. Unlike before, where just a bit of sugar would put you back, treating yourself occasionally will likely not have the same effects and you can likely splurge occasionally. However, you must be very mindful to not fall completely off the wagon and end up back in a sugar-dependent lifestyle. In doing so, you'll simply be wasting all of the progress you made during your sugar detox.

Detoxing from sugar is a trend that many people are considering. It can have great benefits on your mind and body, including your physique and how you feel on a daily basis. Keep in mind the information here, to have a better understanding of how your body handles a sugar detox.

CHAPTER 5- HOW TO EAT RIGHT WHILE ON A SUGAR DETOX

Trying a sugar detox can be both challenging and exciting. If you have a high blood sugar level, suffer from diabetes, or just want to lose weight, a sugar detox can be the answer to all your problems. The detox helps people fix their blood sugar levels and stop you from craving sweets all the time. Sugar is one of the worst things you can stuff into your body because consuming too much sugar is associated with many kinds of diseases. If you have an extreme weakness for baked goodies or something sweet and you can eat a whole batch of cookies in one seating, then a sugar detox is your best bet.

A sugar detox can last from three days to 21 days. Some people claim that a 3-day sugar detox is enough to kick the habit of eating sugary foods mindlessly and stop you from craving sweet goodies all the time. Aside from diabetes, eating too many sweets can lead to many health complications especially since sugar consumption is the number one reason why people are overweight. Being overweight makes people vulnerable and at-risk to many chronic and deadly diseases. This is one main reason for you to become resolved to eliminate your cravings for sweet foods.

Once you start a sugar detox, it will not be a smooth, pleasant ride. It is more than likely that the first few days are going to be horrible. Like all types of detox methods, your body may enter into some form of shock. In fact, during the first few days, your sweet tooth might even become more intense than ever. Instead of curbing your cravings for sweets, you might even long for sweets every other minute. The best thing to do is to just ride these cravings out and stay focused on your goal. More importantly, eat the right foods that will make you stay committed to your detox plan until you forget how it feels to mindlessly crave for sweets.

The important thing to know about sugar detox is that it is not about eating zero sugar. It is about eating the right type of sugary foods and to avoid eating sweet foods without thinking. Therefore, fruits are good to eat if you are a sugar detox. Fruits can regulate your cravings and will not allow you to lose control if you are thinking about sweets too much.

Of course, too many fruits should be avoided as well. To be sure that you are committing to removing your sugar cravings, you can eat moderate amounts of bananas and blueberries. To kick start your day, you can have lemon water and some oranges. However, if you want to be 100% committed to the detox plan, you can skip on fruits and eat as many vegetables as you want instead.

To make sure you are eating right under this detox plan, make sure to prepare for it. Go grocery shopping ahead of time and stock your fridge only with the foods and snacks you are allowed to eat. You can as many vegetables and proteins as you want when doing this detox. If you love salads and meats, then you can be a happy camper while on this diet. You may find doing the groceries difficult especially if carbohydrates and sugary snacks are your staples. To avoid delaying your detox because you saw something sweet you want to try, avoid the aisles where you know the sweets are located.

If you love sugary drinks such as sodas and juices, go for vegetable juices this time. You might realize that they taste better than you expected and they can be part of your daily routine once you are done with the detox. Check the labels to make sure the sugar content is not high. In fact, the sugar content should be at a bare minimum. Choose the ones that are organic.

Once you stock your fridge full of what you can eat, you can also prepare the food you will eat for three days in advance. If you have already prepared the food you need to eat, you will be less likely to give in to your cravings and relapse on your detox; especially if you can imagine the effort you went through to have all the food prepared. If you are working, bringing your food instead of going to the cafeteria or having lunch with friends are the best ideas to eat right while on a sugar detox. You should avoid seeing the sugary stuff you cannot touch so you will not be tempted to grab some dessert just because your friend cannot finish the cake or pie he or she ordered.

Another way to make sure you are eating right while on a sugar detox is to be mindful of your cravings. It is likely that you will only crave sugary foods when you are bored or stressed. If you are stressed, instead of making a trip to a vending machine to get a soda or a chocolate, try to do something relaxing instead. You can watch a funny video clip and let your stresses flow away.

You can call a friend and talk about your day; even for a minute or two. You feel less stressed and forget the urge to get something sweet. If you are bored, you can also play a game on your phone or do something to forget that you want something sweet. Naturally, if you are in the workplace, you must avoid these activities. Certainly though, you can find something to do aside from eating sweets or drinking soda.

Any type of detox is difficult to do. It takes real effort and commitment. A sugar detox is no different. It may even be more challenging than other types of detox simply because people are so used to mindlessly grabbing snacks that are usually sweet throughout the day. If you remember your reasons for wanting to do this detox, it will be easier to survive and eat right throughout this diet.

CHAPTER 6- WHAT TO DO AFTER A SUGAR DETOX

The traditional understanding about sugar's role as a fuel source has recently been redefined with the latest research. Deoxyribonucleic acid (DNA) the genetic blueprints of life has a backbone comprised of phosphate groups and deoxyribose (alternating sugars), with G, A, T, C (nucleobases) attached to these alternating sugars. What is known is that foreign processed sugar is considered a poison to the body and insulin is required to quickly process incoming sugar molecules.

This process leads to cellular respiration a set of metabolic combustion reactions that changes biochemical energy into ATP (adenosine triphosphate), which also includes the release of unwanted waste products. Cellular respiration is necessary to generate useful energy in the vital support of cellular activity. Through the conversion process, carbohydrates will initially become glucose and may continue onward to become pyruvate and then lactate or in the reverse order – lactate, pyruvate, and then glucose. The last portion in the order arrangement is lactate, which is the most essential and the second most wanted fuel source just after fatty acids. Short and medium chain fatty acids are absorbed by blood cells directly and distributed as fuel for metabolism and muscular contraction.

The mitochondria consume fatty acids to produce ATP through beta oxidation. The heart's major or primary source of energy comes from the oxidation of fatty acids and the secondary source is the oxidation of lactate through exercise or excessive stress. These conditions drive lactate oxidation into becoming the primary source of ATP production. The electron acceptor, an oxidizing agent in general oxidation is O2 (molecular oxygen), which lends to the heart of ATP production. The advantage of focusing primarily on fermented foods and on foods that are high in short or medium chain fatty acids – is the transition to perfect body alignment.

Advanced Glycation End Products (AGEs) and Methanogens Role

The glycation of sugars found in Advanced Glycation End Products supply a large portion of oxidative and peroxidative stress on the body which leads to many degenerative diseases, such as diabetes, arthritis, and atherosclerosis. These compounds are very harmful and are derived from the glycation reaction which is the inclusion of a carbohydrate to protein combination without enzyme involvement. AGEs can advance oxidative damage to cells and are a key factor in age related chronic diseases. AGE's can form inside of the body and outside of the body through the heating or cooking of food. Caramel candy is essentially cooked sugar and when applied in a heating process to apples or pastries, the combination forms AGEs.

Methanogens consume AGEs and produce methane as a byproduct through metabolic anoxic conditions. These microorganisms are classified as archaea and are found in the digestive tracts of humans and animals. They are the main source of DNA hypermethylation which interrupts transcription, preventing certain proteins from forming properly and leads to degenerative diseases. In removing sugar and AGEs, Methanogens will be suppressed unable to release large quantities of methane.

The Lectin and Gluten Defense

Every plant, vegetable and herb has a lectin defense mechanism against bacteria. Gluten is a known lectin and is responsible for inflammation and the common weight gain issues. Lectin in general will cause the blood cells to stick together and is active when consumed – even cooked food will contain active lectin. This defense mechanism searches for sugar receptors and sticks to them to starve bacteria, the only problem with this model is that lectin sticks to the insulin receptors in cells. This is the leading cause of insulin resistance and can only be deactivated though food fermentation. Sugar attracts lectin which leads to a variety of problems.

The Sugar Free Solution

Fermentation is the essential key as it provides lactate that is ready to be utilized and the lectin is deactivated, preventing future problems. Pickles, sauerkraut, and other fermented foods can be found in most grocery stores. It is best to learn the process and there are many books that can be found on food fermentation. Not all lectin is binding, for instance coconut oil has a lectin that does not bind blood cells and is high in medium chain fatty acids that are excellent for the body. Omega fatty acids can be found in Chia seeds and avocado.

Lakanto and Stevia Sweeteners

Lakanto is a non-GMO erythritol combined with the super sweet extract of the luo han guo fruit. The sugar alcohol Erythritol is found grapes, beer, and cheese and has been around for thousands of years in the human diet. Erythritol is unique in that this sugar alcohol is fermented corn sugar. The difference between Erythritol and other sugar alcohols is that Lakanto does not cause gas, bloating, and or diarrhea.

Other sugar alcohols are typically made via hydrogenation verse fermentation, which is the difference. This sugar is excellent for those who have diabetes as it will not raise blood sugar levels and Lakanto tastes like natural sugar. Stevia is also an excellent sweetener and is 100 times stronger tasting than regular sugar. Just replacing regular sugar with a better alternative will prevent many age related issues.

Life after sugar does not have to be very difficult and it can be wonderful to know that balance can be achieved. In creating the perfect strategy, it is best to focus on all foods that are high in omega fatty acids, those with non-binding lectin, and those foods that are fermented. The best fruits can be found with these qualities and they are the avocado and lemon. The lemon for its added benefit of a negative electrical charge that provides cells readily available energy. These foods can help you to build a custom sugar free diet that is fulfilling and provides you with amazing energy.

CHAPTER 7- WHAT ARE SOME FREQUENTLY ASKED QUESTIONS ABOUT THE SUGAR DETOX?

There are all sorts of questions that people ask about the sugar detox. People want to know what it is, how to do it, and what all of the benefits are. Below are some of the top questions about the detox in order to provide more information about it.

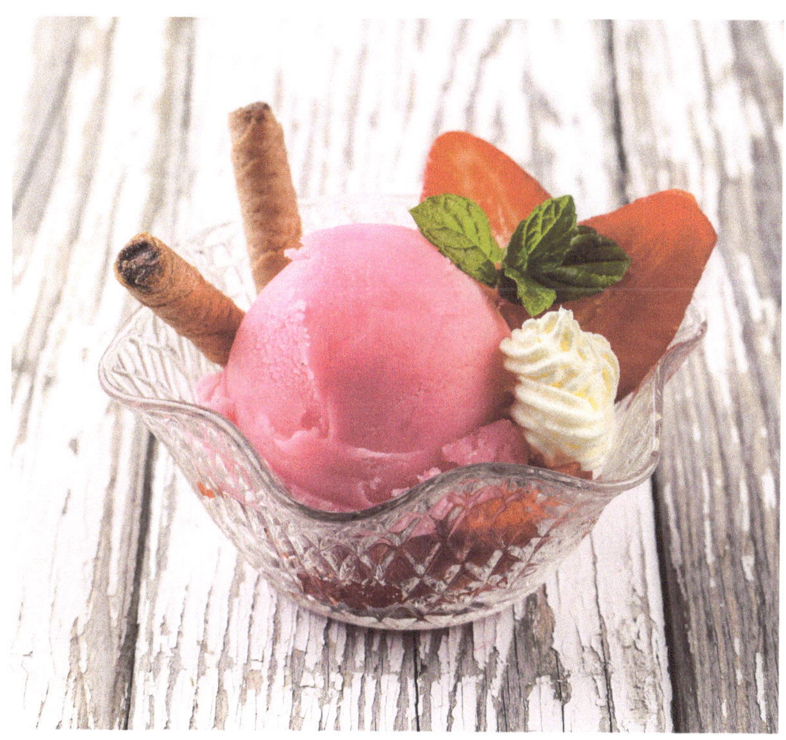

What Is the Sugar Detox?

The Sugar Detox is a form of dieting where sugar is virtually eliminated from the diet in order to provide an array of health benefits.

What's Involved?

There's the 3-day sugar fix where you have to cut out all sugar cold turkey. This means that you aren't going to eat any sugar whatsoever. After the three days are over, you can slowly introduce SOME foods back into your diet as long as they are controlled. The diet consists of four weeks and each week offers some kind of program.

What Kind of Sugar Has To Be Eliminated?

Virtually all kinds of sugar need to be eliminated – including the "hidden" sugars that are found in yogurt, sauces, and things that are commonly labeled "low-fat."

What Is the Recommended Dosage of Sugar?

You should only be consuming 70g of sugar a day for men and 50 grams for women. The problem is that many people are overdoing their consumption by double and triple that amount.

What Are the Health Benefits?

The benefits of the sugar detox diet are that it can help you lose weight, feel better about yourself, and even help you to look younger. You can avoid health problems by dropping weight and the youthful skin that you have been trying to achieve can be obtained.

How Does Sugar Affect Our Appearance

There are collagen and elastin molecules within your skin that help to provide the youthful appearance. When these molecules are damaged, your skin is no longer able to "snap back" and this is going to cause wrinkles. The sugar that goes unprocessed in the bloodstream latches onto protein molecules. These protein-sugar complexes are called AGEs (advanced glycation end products). These can trigger inflammation and break down the tissue in your skin. They are going to attack the collagen and elastin molecules and cause premature aging.

Why Is Sugar Such an Issue?

Sugar is a controlled substance for many because it is being consumed so regularly by Americans. The average American will consume approximately 31 pounds of sugar in a single year. It has led to various health problems including diabetes and obesity.

Why Can't People Control Their Own Sugar

People can control their own sugar, but it all comes down to knowing what to look for – and being able to find the hidden sugars. It is found in virtually everything that you eat and drink. From the coffee that you make in the morning to the crème brulee that you have after dinner, sugar is everywhere. The Centers for Disease Control projected that by 2050, one in three people will have diabetes – and this is because of weight gain and the consumption of sugar.

Could Sugar Really Become a Controlled Substance?

It may come to that because of the various side effects. Since the consumption of sugar is at a high that has never been seen before, it could be controlled similar to that of alcohol and tobacco. There is a group of University of California scientists at the San Francisco campus that have recently recommended that sugar be controlled in the very same manner. This means that it may not be regularly available and that all of the foods that you know and love could be off-limits for good.

What's the Solution?

The solution is to go on The Sugar Detox where you can learn once and for all how to say no to sugar. You don't have to rule out sugar 100 percent from your diet. You do, however, have to learn how to consume it in the right amounts. The first three days are the hardest, but after that, it's going to get a lot easier – especially as you know what to look for and what foods should be avoided.

Why Are the First Three Days the Hardest?

The three days that are the hardest are as a result of quitting cold turkey. It is to help curb the addiction to the sugar. Your body responds to sugar in the same way that it would respond to an addictive drug – it doesn't know how to say no and it makes you want it more and more. By cutting it out entirely for the first three days, you can start to feel better and get onto the path of living a healthier lifestyle.

What Does the Book Include?

The book regarding the Sugar Detox includes information about what sugar does, a guide through the four weeks and what foods can be introduced at which stages, as well as a variety of recipes. Essentially, it is a full guide as to what you can and cannot eat while on the sugar detox diet. Additionally, it provides way to care for your skin and tone your body through an exercise program. When you want to lead a better life, the book will show you how.

Are There Testimonials?

Throughout the book, there are patients and clients that have overcome their sugar habits and now lead a healthier lifestyle where they are no longer ruled by sugar. This can provide you with the willpower to move forward.

ABOUT THE AUTHOR

Amy Zulpa had to really get her research done to figure out what she was going to do to combat the problems that she was having with sugar. She was having a bit of a problem as the excess sugar that she was consuming was starting to affect her health in a big way. When she started to realize how serious it was becoming, she decided to solve the problem quickly as she did not want it to get to a point where she did irreparable damage to her body.

The sugar detox was the last thing that she was going to try before going cold turkey to try and solve the problem. From the success that she had, she decided to share what she had learned with as many persons as possible. Amy is of the belief that a success story is something that should be shared as it can help others to achieve the same positive results.

www.ingramcontent.com/pod-product-compliance
Lightning Source LLC
Chambersburg PA
CBHW042128030726
47599CB00002B/396